Pain Blocking Yoga

Simple Yoga steps to strengthen your mind physically (block out pain) and spiritually (live a lot happier).

Swati Misra

To Vishwas, my husband, who also taught me Yoga. And to my parents, who taught me so much about life.

Table of Content

Read This First

This book uses yoga techniques to help users strengthen their minds. The steps described are mild and generally easy for people to follow - for example techniques for meditation and breathing exercises. However, please note that the process described here does not supersede any advice from your doctor. If you have a history of breathing difficulties, head-aches, sinus problems, lung infections or any other serious or persistent medical issues, please consult your doctor before following the advise of this book. Also, please stop using the book advice if you find that your breathing or heartbeat or any part of your body is discomforted while following the steps described here. While we believe that the book advises simple exercises that should not cause any harm, if you sense that they may be harming you, you should stop using the book and immediately consult your doctor.

A Quick Overview

This book comprises simple instructions in three stages. The first stage, "Prepare", sets the foundation by listing basic building blocks that need to be in place such as healthy eating, exercise, sleep, as well as simple breathing exercises. The Second stage, "Develop the basic skill", comprises instructions to help reach a level where the mind is strengthened to block out pain. Success in this stage will come with dedication, persistence, and regular practice. The Third Stage, "Extend the Skill", shows how the very same mind control skill may be used to put us in a lasting state of peace and happiness. This third stage provides an important insight: that we can use the same yoga techniques to block out physical pain as well as to bring peace and happiness to our minds. The larger point here is that yoga is as much about strengthening our minds as it is about keeping our bodies healthy.

Expect this to be a journey

Please remember that the yoga instructions here will take you through a journey. And as with any journey, your reaching a destination depends on whether you are moving in the right direction and the speed with which you move. Frequent, regular, and persistent effort should generally get you there in a matter of a few months- even weeks. Sporadic, irregular effort may not get you there even after years. The eventual destination is very, very rewarding and worth the effort. Once we achieve a measure of control over our minds, you would wonder how you lived without such control. Good luck and happy journey. It helps a lot if you try and enjoy this as a process of discovery.

Prepare

In this phase, you will be advised to take some preparatory steps. These steps relate to basic health advise on food, sleeping, and exercise, as well as learning some basic breathing techniques. Consult your doctor in case you have a serious or potentially painful medical condition that may prevent you from following any suggestions here (when in doubt, please consult your doctor). Your doctor's advice should take precedence over the advice here.

The Basics

Healthy Eating

Ideally, your diet should be vegetarian with enough daily servings of fruits, salads, and vegetables that are high on fiber. There is enough advise on good vegetarian eating out there, so it will not be covered here. If you are in doubt, we encourage you to research this over Internet and arrive at a good diet plan for yourself. Non-vegetarian food (meat) may be less conducive to yogic advancement and should be avoided (especially red meat). Spicy food should be avoided as well. Also cut down on sugar and processed carbohydrates. They are not stable sources of energy and do not help when one embarks on yogic strengthening of mind.

Get Enough Sleep

Managing your time to get a minimum of 7-8 hours of sleep daily is important.

Yogic advance is impossible if you are not getting enough sleep.

Exercise Daily

Please ensure that you are getting a good, regular, aerobic work-out. If you would like to keep this simple, a minimum of 30 minutes of daily, moderate-speed walking would be good.

Healthy Breathing

The advice so far is seen as standard stuff for healthy living. It is important, nonetheless, to lay the foundations for yogic advancement. Now, let's start getting into more targeted exercise.

Breathing is a very strong tool for yogic mind control. Yet, we rarely realize its potential. See if you can notice this going forward: you are likely to lose control over your breath just as you get angry. Yogic science sees anger as a loss of control over the mind. And it teaches us that if we can retain control over our breath (in a specific manner), then we can retain control over our minds. Pain and happiness can also be similarly controlled - as you will discover in this journey.

As a first step, we suggest you start with "Breathing Exercise 1" described below. As you follow it, please remember that the ultimate objective is to calm and control our minds. So, we advise you to seek to put your mind at peace during this exercise and the ones that follow.

Breathing Exercise 1

Here is a simple breathing exercise that will serve as a foundation for your yoga exercises. Please read the full section before you start.

Start with breathing out completely (push air out of your lungs only to the point where you remain comfortable).

Step 1: Expand your stomach to breath in. Count 1.

Step 2: Expand your chest to continue breathing in. Count 2.

Step 3: Contract your chest to breathe out. Count 1.

Step 4: Contract your stomach to continue breathing out. Count 2.

Now go back to "Step 1".

Breathe easy while doing this exercise. Do not strain yourself. Do not try and stuff your lungs with air. And do not try and get all the air out of them either. While breathing in and out, expand and contract only up to the point you are comfortable. You can do this breathing exercise any time in the day. And you need to be able to do this fluently and easily before you move to the next exercise.

In the next exercise, we use the term "2-step breathing in" to describe first breathing in through stomach expansion and then chest expansion and "2-step breathing out" as chest contraction and then stomach contraction.

Please practice the "Breathing Exercise 1" and become fluent with it before moving on to the "Breathing Exercise 2". This fluency may need a few days of practice.

Breathing Exercise 2

We will describe a breathing exercise here that we recommend you to do for around 10 minutes each day. The exercise must be done in the morning before eating anything (you may drink moderate amount of water (around 1 glass) before it - if you like. We recommend that this exercise become a become a permanent part of your daily routine.

Please read all the sections below carefully to understand the exercise before you try and follow them. Remember the 2-step breathing in and 2-step breathing out you learnt in "Breathing Exercise 1". These would be used here.

Preparing For The Exercise

Prep Step 1: sit in a posture that is comfortable for you and keeps your back straight. Ideally, you would be sitting on a broad, flat surface that is not a chair and not too soft (would make you slouch) or too hard (would make you uncomfortable). A firm bed or mattress would be ideal.

Prep Step 2: close your eyes and breathe calmly for around 5 minutes. You should aim to calm your mind and steady your breathing. Follow the breathing you learned in "Breathing Exercise 1".

Prep Step 3: after 5 minutes of calm breathing, raise your right hand (or if you prefer, the left hand) to your nose.

Prep Step 4: breathe out up to a point where you have exhaled the air in your lungs but do not strain yourself. Now move on to the exercise steps described in the next section.

The Exercise

Start with exhaling (breathing out).

Step 1: Close the left nostril and breathe in through the right nostril. Inhale deeply till you have filled up your lungs. Do not fill them up too much. One way some people do this is to imagine that the air has filled up their chest up to their neck and then stop inhaling. The breathing in should be at a relaxed, normal speed. Use the "2-step breathing in" you learnt earlier.

Step 2: Close your right nostril and open your left nostril. Now breathe out through the left nostril. Breathe out only up to the point you are comfortable. Do not strain yourself. Use the "2-step breathing out" you learnt earlier.

Step 3: Now breathe in through the left nostril using the "2-step breathing in process" while keeping the right nostril closed.

Step 4: Close the left nostril, open the right nostril and breathe our through the right nostril using "2-step breathing in".

Go back to Step 1- to the point where in through the right nostril. Repeat the cycle for 10 minutes. Feel free to switch hands if you get tired.

In Summary, breathe in through the right nostril, close it, breathe out through the left, breathe in through the left, close it, breathe out through the right and then repeat from breathing in through the right.

Caution: Do not do this exercise for more than 15 minutes at a stretch. Long sessions of this exercise need to be done under close supervision by yoga experts. And if you have any serious medical condition, especially related to breathing or heart, please consult your doctor and seek permission before doing these exercises. Do not do this exercise against medical advice.

A Few Points to Note On This Exercise

1. Although this exercise is gentle, you should remain careful. If you feel any discomfort while doing the above exercise, stop at once and consult a doctor. Do not do this exercise if you feel any discomfort or against medical advice.

2. People often complain that they have only one nostril available for breathing and the other one appears blocked. Here are some suggestions to get around this problem: Firstly, do some moderate exercises for 10-15 minutes before the breathing exercise. This could be walking at a moderate speed or doing simple yoga

positions. Such activity should open up the nostril at least partially. Secondly, while breathing in and out of the blocked nostril, force air in and out gently. Do not use a lot of force to push the air through the nostril. Be gentle. Despite your attempts, if one nostril remains stubbornly blocked, look for an alternative time when you can do this exercise.

3. This breathing exercise has psychological benefits. People generally report lesser incidences of cold, cough and other breathing ailments once they start on this. And they generally feel that the exercise has a calming impact on their minds and also make them more alert. This exercise also (after a few weeks / months) makes sure that both your nostrils remain open for most of the time during the day.

4. This exercise is a recommended breathing technique within yoga called "Pranayaam". There are multiple

variations of "Pranayaam" that address different physiological requirements. We encourage you to look them up on the Internet and see how these help people live better lives.

Moving To The Next Section

You can start on the next section even as you are learning the "Breathing Exercise 2".

Develop The Basic Skill

This section will now describe to you three activities that you will need to keep practicing.

1. A specific type of meditation that you need to do at least once daily.

2. A specific way by which you need to start eating your food.

3. How to start blocking out pain when it strikes.

You do not need to follow the section recommendations one-at-a-time. In fact, we recommend that you start performing all of them daily.

The objective of this section is to help you start controlling your mind. By "controlling your mind" we mean, "controlling how your senses impact your mind". For example, pain is a sense perception. If you would like to control how your mind senses pain, you need to start controlling how your mind senses the signals it gets from your body. Once you successfully advance through these exercises, you should learn to "develop a switch" in your mind that you can turn off – when you want to block your senses.

Special Meditation Exercise

We will now develop specific skills to strengthen our minds. This exercise helps focus the mind.

As in the breathing exercise, sit in a posture that is comfortable for you and keeps your back straight. As earlier, you should be sitting on a broad, flat surface that is not a chair and not too soft or too hard. A firm bed or mattress would be ideal. Half close your eyes and focus them on something in front, for example, a wall. The eyes should remain relaxed. Remember to keep the focus soft and not strain your eyes. If you prefer, you could focus on something more distant (a more distant focus makes the exercise less effective). Either way, make sure your eyes are relaxed and not strained.

Now bring your attention to your forehead- specifically the region between your eyebrows. This focusing of attention on the forehead is crucial. The best way to get this done is to imagine your entire existence rising up and getting into the region between your eyebrows. Those who believe in God should try to feel His presence there and may find this meditation very rewarding. It provides a sense of merging one's existence with God. Others can imagine something that they consider uplifting and infinitely stronger than themselves over there (some like to imagine a bight light that they associate with goodness). Either way, maintain your attention between your eyebrows and try and hold it there for 15-20 minutes. It is common for the mind to drift at this time. When it does, bring it back. And be patient.

When you start this exercise you should ideally breathe with the "Breathing

Exercise 1" technique. Each breath (incoming and outgoing) is surrendered to the entity you are imagining to be present between your eyebrows.

As you advance, you will feel deeply relaxed and that your breathing becomes shallow. Only a very slight amount of air comes in (feel it being offered to what you're imagining between your eyebrows) and only a slight amount goes out- again being offered to the same entity. This is not a cause for alarm. Continue unless you feel any physical discomfort. This subtle sense of gentle breathing is one of the foundations of your mind control. As you get into this state, imagine your whole existence shrinking into the space between your eyebrows. You, in effect, surrender yourself to the higher entity you imagine here. This process of surrendering is important and will be used later. Practice this surrender again and again.

After you start this meditation, when you separately do "Breathing Exercise 2", you should feel the incoming air going into the space between your eyebrows and the outgoing air originating from your from the space between the eyebrows- going out. Your breathing during the "Breathing Exercise 2" should remain deep and should not turn shallow. It is during this meditation only that your breathing automatically becomes relaxed and shallow and you allow it to do so.

A Note on Relaxing Your Mind

Relaxing your mind and keeping it that way is a pleasure we want you to discover. Practice this relaxation meditation technique whenever you are free. Beware that doing so sometimes puts you to sleep. From a yoga standpoint, that is not harmful. But, please ensure that you don't practice this meditation when you need to be very alert, for example while driving a car.

Suggestion: Next time you are free, try this relaxation technique instead of pulling out your smartphone!

Eating Exercise!

Now is when you try and control how your senses touch your mind. Food has a powerful sensory impact on virtually every mind. When you start controlling its impact on your mind, you learn the technique that is needed to block out pain (and also, as you will learn later, a way to keep your mind happy throughout). Your doing this exercise does not imply that you will stop enjoying the taste of food once you perfect this technique. Like any muscle in your control, this ability to control senses will be there for you to use when you choose. And like any muscle, it will be strengthened with more use and practice.

The Exercise

Here's what we recommend: Make sure you are sitting in a posture where your back is erect while eating. Ideally, you should be eating healthy food that you also like. The food must not be spicy. Once you place the food in your mouth and start chewing it, its taste reaches your mind. At this time, use the technique you learnt during meditation and try and surrender this taste to the same entity you imagined during the meditation. You were surrendering your outgoing breath during the meditation. You surrender the taste during eating in exactly the same way. Keep practicing.

Points To Note About The Eating Exercise

This exercise is best done alone. Although eating is now a social activity, we do recommend that you find time to eat in silence and in a manner that allows you to concentrate while doing this exercise.

Typically, people are only able to do this exercise well for a few gulps of food and not all. This is not an easy exercise, as the mind tends to get distracted. Be patient and bring it back each time.

When you eat as described above, you begin to take control of how your senses impact your mind. Soon, you will reach a point where you feel that the impact of the taste reduces and this taste is surrendered to the entity you imagine. And, as we describe in the next section, this is the same technique you use to block out physical pain. In the section after that we will touch upon how this skill can be extended to keep our minds happy and at peace.

A Note For The Religious Reader

Offering food to God is very highly regarded across most religions. One way to do so is to offer the taste of the food to God – in the manner described above. When done well, religious readers will actually feel as though the food is being sent up to God (situated between eyebrows) and not down to the stomach. Although that is not physically happening, this can be a very satisfying experience for the religiously minded.

Pain Blocking Exercise

We will now describe how you can start blocking out pain.

Before we start, please note the following: do not inflict pain on yourself to practice pain-blocking. Such infliction of pain is perverse and must not be done. Your normal life will normally provide you with opportunities to practice pain blocking. You need to summon your pain blocking skills at these times.

When pain strikes...

When pain strikes, you need to get your mind back to the state you are in when you are meditating and surrendering yourself to the entity between your eyebrows. While a part of your body pains, you need to concentrate (as you do in meditation) and imagine yourself shrinking completely into the space between your eyebrows. As you surrender yourself to this higher entity, the pain separates from you. You have then withdrawn into your forehead while the pain is elsewhere in the body. The pain sensation is blocked just as the sensation of taste is blocked during eating. That's it. It's as simple as that. The discomfort from the pain stops although you may continue to feel it in a different manner. For example, if the pain was in the thigh, the discomfort goes away and is replaced by a feeling of carrying something heavy in your pocket. You can feel an object's presence there but it does not cause you pain.

Keep Practicing

Even as you may feel that you are getting more and more advanced on this path, you need to keep practicing. As you practice this pain blocking, you may initially face greater success when the pain originates from certain areas like the hands and feet and a less success when it originates from certain other areas like above the neck. As you practice the eating and meditation suggested here, you begin to block out the more challenging pain as well.

Extend The Skill

Now you know that we are using a very similar technique during the meditation, eating, and blocking out pain. This makes things simple. We need to do the same thing over and over to meditate well and to block out pain. In this section we will describe how the same exact technique may be used to raise our general level of happiness and peace. Pain blocking is one way to apply your new skill. Another, even better, book is to raise the level of happiness of your mind on a permanent basis. We will describe how this may be done.

Deepening The Skill

You need to consciously summon your pain blocking skill each time you experience pain. Normally, the pain is unexpected and sudden. The mind is unprepared and not on guard. Once you experience the pain, your mind is ready and can consciously summon the pain blocking technique to prevent the sensation of pain from disturbing it. After some time (usually several months of practice) the summoning of pain blocking technique happens automatically. Once developed, the mind still remains unprepared but does not wait for you to consciously summon the technique. The skill is summoned as a reflex (automatic reaction) to pain. When you reach this stage, you experience pain only in the first split second when the mind is unprepared. As soon as pain strikes, the mind blocks it. Reaching this level of mental strength is supremely satisfying. But don't get complacent, you can and must keep strengthening this skill. Also note that this pain blocking happens when pain presents itself as a "target" for at least a few seconds. Flashes of pain are not easily blocked as they subside before you summon this skill.

Use the skill to be Always Happy

The same skill of blocking out pain may be used to block out all the unease, tension, and even anger that one may feel at any time. Just as pain is blocked out, a person may block out the negative energy that prevents our mind from enjoying every moment of this life. Yes, that is right, we can enjoy each moment if we consciously start applying the technique we have learnt here. And the book is the same- to block out negative energy and to realize happiness. Here's how it works: if you feel a negative emotion such as anger, you can leave it behind in your body (like you leave pain) as you surrender yourself to the infinite, positive energy between your eyebrows. Alternatively, in the normal course of your day, when can imagine yourself giving yourself (surrendering) into that entity and, in return, feel a sense of deep happiness and contentment. The same exact technique works in both cases. Soon, you should start living in a higher level of existence where your spend more and more of your time in direct connect with the entity that brings you peace and happiness. Repeating for emphasis: For those who are religious, imagining God or a religious artifact or a holy light to be that entity is deeply satisfying. For others, it may help to imagine the entity as something infinite, much greater than themselves, and embodying all that they deem good and positive.

Endnote

Reducing the impact of pain on your body and being in a constant state of happiness effectively raise the level of our living to another plane. We wish you every success and you embark on this journey. As you progress, we recommend that you continue to practice a few exercises:

1. Breathing Exercise 2.

2. Eating – as suggested here.

3. Meditation – as suggested here. Also try and replicate this state of peace during your daily routine.

On Yoga

The techniques described here are from the science of Yoga. And Yoga focuses on the following:

1. Stillness. Even as your body engages in activity, search for stillness and peace in your mind.

2. Search for happiness within: According to Yogic Literature, a life that is spent only in pursuit of sense pleasures is a life spent in vain. Instead of having our senses look outside, Yoga helps us find happiness within. The outside world can keep changing. But the stillness inside can be a source of permanent joy.

3. Service: reduced reliance on our senses for happiness is a stepping-stone towards helping others who are less fortunate than ourselves (all living beings- not just humans).

We encourage you to continue exploring Yoga – both of body and mind. Keep practicing. And enjoy the journey to discover your mind.